SETS IN THE CITY

Transform Your Body As A City Professional

Vlad Galbavy

Published In 2016

To all my clients and all the people in the City chasing their goals.

"This book is like exploring the Great Wall of China journey, once you start reading it inspires you to explore your body and mind capabilities."

Alvin Wong,
Barrister

"A clear outline of how to clarify your goals, stay focused and lead you to what you want to achieve."

Gareth Jones,
Business Analyst at Volbroker

"Reading this reminds me of all the reasons I got into fitness in the first place. Take time and refocus your energies. A great book for The City professional."

Patrick Stapleton,
Key Account Manager at Decision Resources Group

TABLE OF CONTENTS

V. Winners hall

Why City people go to gym and train / Patrick's success / James' success / Chris' success / Gareth's success / Rob's success / A success wrap up / It's not a choice it's a necessity / The opportunity cost / This is what I promote / Halo effect / What are you waiting for? / Call me maybe?

Acknowledgements

Thanks to my early mentor and great friend Tim Robinson. A lot of the views shared in this book evolved from our never-ending discussions about the nature of our work.

Thank you to all people that participated in the creation of this book:
Janice who's perfected my original manuscript; Leo, Sunny and Tim for consulting the ideas in this book; to my clients who offered me the early feedback, and I also wish to give credits to my client Jason for the genius book title.

Thanks to all my clients who committed themselves to changing their bodies and improving their lives for the better.

Introduction

Dear Reader,

Sets In The City is my second book after publishing my first book Body Aesthetics in 2013. I've come a long way since then and while Body Aesthetics was about the know-how and the necessary training and nutritional guidance to transform your body, Sets In The City is about making you follow through as a busy person with a packed daily agenda. The reason I wrote this book is to establish the credibility of body coaching as a performance booster for professionals and to entertain you at the same time. I expect you to read this book because it has good potential not only to help you achieve your optimal physique but to get you promoted, attract a partner, make you excel in your business and simply take your life to a completely new level. The stories in this book are mostly of male clients but they're perfectly relevant to both men and women. So realising you're busy enough, let's get right into it. The book is fairly short and divided into manageable chapters so you can finish and get to understand it within 30 minutes, which is a ride home on a tube.

Enjoy!
Vlad Galbavy
vlad@setsinthecity.co.uk
www.setsinthecity.co.uk

I. WHY IS THIS BOOK IMPORTANT TO YOU?

Living in The City, hustling in your job, going to client lunches and dinners, meeting loads of people, having fun and boozing every now and then, all of these have a major effect on your body, so this book is for you if your lifestyle leaves you tired, your body doesn't look the way you want and you're not feeling that healthy as a result. Now in case you skipped the introduction there are 3 major points I want to make with this book. There is a reason why you want to work on your body, you need to see fitness from the perspective of your core values and you need to take a unique approach as you work and live in The City. That's why this book holds the ultimate key to fitness success within a busy environment. The information this book contains has helped various people from CEOs to VCs who have transformed their bodies and as a result their lives and it will allow you to reach your maximum potential for both your body and your mind too. It is meant to psych you up for your training and healthy eating because only those who are highly motivated will ever manage to have a fit and healthy looking body leading to high performance levels in all areas of their lives. The testimonial to this sentence are all the people mentioned in this book who transformed their bodies because they were consistently working on themselves and investing their time in their health and appearance while keeping their mindset on the absolute top level. In all their cases their whole lives improved together with their bodies. And it wasn't because of the tools that I gave them because the tools are never going to do it for you, only you are, and for that you need to be psyched up. And that's what I'm trying to accomplish with this book.

FITNESS ECONOMICS 101

Before I say anything else there is one absolutely crucial thing we need to establish. While you might think you're saving yourself time and energy for doing things you deem more important by not training and not eating properly, the truth is that training and proper eating will raise your performance to the top level. And we all know the City is all about hustling so your performance level is important. Now, you work in the City as a business person so what I'm talking about is that taking care of your body so you can perform on a higher level and perhaps experience some sort of a breakthrough somewhere else as well, is the same as spending 2 hours with a client for lunch because of the potential deal coming out of the good relationship. I'm talking about some solid progress with your body that so few people actually manage to achieve consistently, because if you're like most of the people then your progress is probably very slow or non-existent. And that's bad because you need to keep your hustle on. Look, if you've made no progress lately then you're missing out big time. What you're missing on I don't know. But this book will help you discover it together with your absolute pay-off for keeping your body making solid progress and taking a great care of it. So let's get into the juicy stuff.

JASON'S STORY

Jason's lost 9kg of bodyweight in 35 days and it all starts with him saying he hates exercise. Quite a bizarre statement for such a success but he's got his reasons and that's clearly one of the most important things on this journey. He's already had 3 different PT's but not too much progress, which is a shame because he's been putting the time into it. So why has he made such a killing now and hardly any progress before? He's a CEO of a publicly traded company so his ability has never been the problem. What's the difference then? What's going on in his mind? What has made him work out regularly, push himself really hard, be disciplined with his food and do it every single day for a month, two or more?

The answer lies in this book and the answer to this is the answer to you making a difference in whatever you want to do with your body. And it's not about knowing what to do. Most of the people know what to do and they don't do it anyway. It's also not about being weak-minded. All my clients work in the City, which is basically a collection of some of the smartest and most determined people in the whole world so ability is definitely not the problem. Understanding what to do and being disciplined and performing on a high level are common factors here. Being able to do this for your fitness and your body seems to be a mystery for whatever reason though. If it sounds familiar and you feel like you're a part of it most of the time, welcome to the City of London.

FITNESS LIFE IN THE CITY OF LONDON

People come to work in the City for one reason. They want to make a killing and they want to play their lives on a top level. High performance work environment, high social life expectations and the desire to do more are all in their DNA. And the chances are that you're a part of it too. Working long hours, running client meetings, spending lot of time on the phone, chasing deals, shaking hands, following your vision and let's not forget about your social life, family life and personal goals as well. Quite a demand. Fortunately enough, most of the people now understand that your mental performance is directly linked to your fitness and wellbeing and so they make some effort to come to the gym and do something with their bodies. Having an optimal hormonal balance, stabilised blood sugar levels, proper blood flow, improved self-image, increased confidence and imposing a top standard perception when meeting people face-to-face are some of the things that determine the outcome of your micro-situations like meetings, decision-making, simple work tasks or anything else in your life, whether it's dating, going on a new adventure, setting up a new business or expanding your circle of influence. Just imagine interacting with people in your top potential body. Do you think it would make any difference? Without realising it a lot of these outcomes and events are influenced by what's going on with and inside your body, and by influencing it you can tip the odds of you becoming a superstar in whatever you do in your life to your side. And that's what I want to accomplish with this book. It gets quite deep.

UNLOCKING YOUR ACHIEVEMENT POTENTIAL

The purpose of this book is to get you into your zone. Imagine things being effortless. When was the last time you felt like that? What made you feel like it? How did it affect everything you did at that time? How did it affect people around you? Think about it. As a professional working in the City you might not see your body as one of the priorities. But it can definitely get you to the state of maximum performance and affect all your priorities on a very profound level. You might be focused on your earning potential, personal growth, family, friends or leisure pursuits but if you're not working on your body you won't be fully able to get what might seemingly be within your reach. It affects everything and I've seen it too many times now for it not to be true. People getting promoted, starting new businesses, starting new relationships, expanding their family, reaching some new personal goals and so on. Just because they got to the top of their game with their body and started making progress. And it spreads out. You're not just working on your body and pleasing your ego. You're literally unlocking doors to some unknown territories and expanding to a new space like never before. Your plans are already crafted in the back of your mind. You just need something to enable yourself to go and get it all.

MY STORY

I came to the City in early 2014 and my main goal was to establish my network with people of high ambition through body coaching and positive mindset maintenance. I imagined this to be the highway to my personal wealth and 2 years later now I know it was one of the best decisions I could have made because I've managed to surround myself with the people of high consciousness, high ambition, high expectations and high standards, which in turn stimulates my mind to grow in many new ways. Moreover, when I first came here I came with an expertise and insights into bocy transformation only but what I perfected over time is the abili:y to understand all the motivations of people in the City and can comfortably say that I'm now not only able to change people's bodies but also to create a massive impact on other areas of their lives as a result of the ripple effect of my coaching. And that's infectious. Your mind stays charged up for such a long time that the outcomes all around you are, not surprisingly, very positive. And that's what I do in the City.

WHY SHOULD YOU LISTEN TO ME?

The main core of what I do is coaching, which means I facilitate behavioural change. I've delivered over 1500 hours of coaching with individual clients who are all City professionals in a little less than 2 years bringing them absolutely top results in the industry. I've been able to make people follow through on their promises through busy times they faced in their business or personal lives and I've been able to keep people accountable to themselves when they experienced some setbacks and managed to do all of this consistently. Now the reason I'm saying that, is that I want to make sure you know everything in this book has been tested repeatedly and is not just a theory but an observation of many real life cases which I've been able to prove with my clients.

WHO DO I NORMALLY WORK WITH?

If you've never met any of my clients it's not too hard to imagine them. They're normally brokers, vice-presidents, CEOs, top executives, entrepreneurs, VCs, sales people, business analysts, doctors, lawyers, consultants and technology people between 25 and 55 years old, with most of them being around 30. They're all great to hang out with and understand the importance of their bodies. More importantly, they also now understand the depth of their bodies' influence on everything they do in life. And that's how they treat it as well. For them, it's not about lifting weights and running or cycling with some high intensity training sessions so they could get defined or look incredibly fit. That's a given. For them it's about directly going after what they know they should be going after because that's who they are. Not only when it comes to their bodies but everything. They're all in touch with their inner selves and experience an increased sense of self-worth.

THE DRIVE

They understand their game. And if you want to improve your body then you might want to tighten up yours too. Have you ever wondered why people come to the gym and work hard on themselves? Do they just want to look and feel better and is that why they come and that's it? Or is there a deeper incentive behind that? What do you think drives everyone? Everyone's got their own game in their head. While some people come to gym to get into shape, experience improved health and get rid of their insecurities, some people are on that level already and got more advanced goals and incentives like optimising their hormones for improved performance or reaching the best shape of their lives for whatever reason they define. It's all individual. Lots of times people don't even know what drives them because it's all driven subconsciously and they've never thought about it so they can't define it properly. Everyone's trying to reach something more valuable than just a change in their body. Everyone's stepping their game up. So let's try to step yours up too.

WHAT DO YOU WANT TO ACHIEVE?

The first question I ask when I consult people is what they want to achieve. This is the one thing that needs to be defined well because this is how you measure your progress. And progress equals happiness. About 80% of people focus mainly on their looks while the rest care mostly about their fitness and wellbeing. Which one do you focus on? What's important to you? Make sure you define it properly. Sometimes people tell me they want to get fitter, we talk for 5 minutes and I actually find out they want to look sharp in meetings so they want to get into proper shape. There's nothing wrong about wanting to look great. It's what the most of us in the City of London want anyway. Just be aware of it. Most people keep coming to the gym stuck in a routine on autopilot not being mindful about what they're doing. And that's when you're done. So ask yourself a question. What do you want to achieve with your body?

HOW HAS YOUR PROGRESS BEEN LATELY?

If you're like most people then probably very slow or non-existent. But again, if you've made no progress at all then you're missing out big time. I had a client who crafted a sound business plan for a very niche market at the time of his fastest progress and also bought another company into his portfolio but then when we stopped training and his goals became more vague, his progress gradually slowed down and he also slowly let go of the plan for his new company and perhaps missed out on a great business opportunity as well. If you're making progress in the gym you're most likely to be making progress somewhere else as well because your game is strong. If you're not making any progress though and your mind is not there either I guarantee you you're missing out on some big things outside of the gym because of the lack of your hormonal support, the strength of your vision, or whatever training brings with it. You're simply not as hungry as you could potentially be and spending the best years of your life hustling in the City without being hungry could as well be spent enjoying yourself somewhere else.

HOW IMPORTANT IS THIS TO YOU?

"I'm getting married in a few months so it's really important to me." And I've never seen the guy in the gym again... I still remember the look in his eyes. They reflected the way he really felt about changing his body. Moving to London 2 years before meeting me, getting straight into the busy City life, finding the girl of his dreams and putting on so much weight that his health was in danger now, his eyes reflected a deep desire to change something but at the same time a fear saying it was never going to happen. He must have felt the price to pay was way too high compared to his expectations. He expected to change something but to still stay in his comfort zone. Imagine the pain of looking at his wedding pictures a few years from now. If you know you owe something to your body, then do it. Don't make your next promotion the highest priority. It will come. Your improved hormonal balance will get you there anyway. Invest in your body instead. If staying in your comfort zone is what you want, then you might not reach your next promotion anyway and you won't even be fitter or better looking either. The only way you can change your body is by making it a priority. It doesn't need to be the number one priority if you can communicate it to yourself from the perspective of your actual priorities but it needs to have a firm place on your agenda.

DO YOU BELIEVE YOUR CHANGE IS POSSIBLE?

I've once been told by one of my clients that he actually didn't initially believe he could change anything about his body. And he said it after going from 76kg to 70kg and reducing his body fat by 5%. Quite a surprising statement as I see people transforming their bodies very often as it's my job but I get it. Lots of people decide to go and change something about their bodies and fail. Lack of knowledge or lack of discipline or they just don't follow through. Then you get 5 people you know talking about their failures and the generalization is out. What's important though is what you take out of it. You're a City professional. You're not working in the City by chance. You're next level. You understand the rules. Give something first and you get something back. It never fails. So do you believe it's possible for you to change your body? Can you see yourself in your best shape? It's so important to be able to do that. Stretch your imagination. See yourself in your new body. I hope you can see it because next I want you to think about your environment. Are you making more money as well? Maybe a different social circle? Surrounded by opportunities? Is your partner proud of you? Or your dating just got to another level? The more you can use your imagination the more you'll see the connection between transforming your body and excelling in whatever you want to.

HOW ACHIEVABLE IS YOUR CHANGE?

I once met this middle-aged accountant who was really interested in working out with me and so we set up a session and worked out together for half an hour. Paul loved it so we sat down to see if it could work for him and his long-term goal, which was to lose his beer belly and work on rotational movements to improve his game in golf. I found out what he was about and what he wanted and proposed a plan. He said he was really interested - until he learned he would need to cut down on boozing. You should have seen the smile on his face. Priceless. He said he was having 10 pints a day, at least 4 days a week, and there was no way he would stop doing it right now. It was a choice he made. I've seen people losing weight while drinking although drinking only at certain times so it wouldn't stop their progress. In Paul's case though, the change was not achievable. Not because of his ability but because of his desire to stay in his comfort zone. The power of choice is a serious thing. If you set your goal properly your change is always achievable. The question is how much of that change you will allow through your mindset.

A QUESTION OF INTEGRITY

The last thing I want to ask you is this. How important is it for you to actually do something about something that's important to you? Think about it. A second ago you defined what you wanted to achieve with your body. Now follow up on it. You're making decisions like these every day in different areas of your life. Make the same choice with fitness as well. Your body is not the last thing to take care of but the first. I know you're travelling for business, commuting to work, doing client entertainment, working long hours, having a busy social life and hustling all the time. But find 3 to 5 hours a week for one of the most important things you possess – your body. Otherwise you're missing out, not maximising. Your body comes first. A fit body makes you feel more energetic and confident and that influences a great deal of things. It gives you an edge. You know what you need to do with your body so do it. This book is about you doing what you know you should do and not turning yourself against yourself. There are way too many people who do that already because it's comfortable and easy. You're not one of them. Otherwise you wouldn't be working here. This is the next level. The second chapter will prove it as well. It will help you find your reason and perhaps put you into the rabbit hole as you'll start realising what the real reason your body needs attention actually is.

II. You need to have a reason

NICHOLAS' STORY

When I first met Nicholas I wasn't really equipped enough to find out what his reason for training was and he couldn't really define it clearly enough on the spot himself. It put me into the world of assumptions, which as you know is not a 100% hit all the time but I accepted it as a lesson. I focused on the training instead and hoped Nicholas would be inspired to push outside of our sessions as well. But his results were slower than I wanted them to be. So it made me think a lot on a daily basis because he had the right tools but literally zero coaching from me apart from all the food and exercise information. I had no firm ground to base my coaching on and I didn't know what to do with it. I felt I was failing but wasn't willing to give up. I spoke with some people and thought about it quite regularly until about 3 months after I first realised I had to do something when I cracked it all and finally managed to get him to commit week after week. Soon enough he made his breakthrough and made more progress than ever before. I think it was more of an accident than a result of my skills back then but it taught me a very important lesson. All action starts with a reason that will empower you towards your goals. And that's why I always make sure both you and I understand your reasons for doing this and that's what this chapter is about.

ASK WHY

So the important thing to realise is that behind everything you want there's a need. And the need can be translated into a reason. And that's incredibly important because that's where the power is. Without knowing why you want to change your body, your goal doesn't matter, your programme doesn't matter, your food doesn't matter and your vision doesn't matter. It's extremely crucial to pay attention to this. Why are you trying to achieve what you're trying to achieve? What's driving you? With every client that I train it's incredibly important to establish the reason why their goal is important to them. It helps them understand their motivations and focus on achieving their goal and it helps me to coach them effectively so they get what they want no matter what. If they want to hit their goals, I need to understand their drivers. If they want to achieve a 6-pack it doesn't matter that they want to achieve a 6-pack. It's only why they want to have their 6-pack that will help them achieve their results. If your partner makes you feel uncomfortable and you feel insecure about your body, then fine. If you can get in touch with that then that's going to get you your goal. Whether it's something deeper than that and you need to get in touch with it then do it. The point is that you need to explore your reasons, be real about them, understand them and then use them as a force helping you get your results.

WHAT'S YOUR REASON?

People getting married, fighting their insecurities, wanting to appeal to their partner, over-performing their siblings, preventing cardiovascular disease, improving posture, fixing back pain or neck pain, getting some blood circulation after a long day behind the desk, fixing muscle imbalances, improving functionality, managing stress, postponing the signs of aging and a few more stick out as the main reasons. Reasons for people to come down to gym and work hard on themselves are all similar after a while. Every now and then there's someone who's got a different reason but the core of gym-goers share one or more of these main drivers. You obviously have your own. Now the thing is that all my clients with the best results have always been the people who have managed to define their reasons with the most clarity and understood what was at stake for them. The people who had the least clarity had problems making progress and moving on because when the time for them to make choices about food and lifestyle came, they were willing to compromise too much. All the top achievers I've trained with always knew why they wanted it whether consciously or subconsciously, defined it to the detail and hit the jackpot. It's not a coincidence. With everyone else, I work on shifting their mindset so they don't fall behind.

DEPTH WITH CLARITY

In early 2015 I met two people who understood their reasons extremely well - Patrick and James. When I consulted them they told me exactly what was driving them and why they wanted to train. They were so clear that even I was amazed. So much clarity in who they were and what they wanted. And that's what made them excel. When other people started losing their focus they were pushing harder. When other people started making excuses they made commitments. It was such an easy job for me. I told them what to do and made sure their mindset stayed charged up. They were killing it and they loved what they were doing. Their results spoke for themselves. And they weren't alone. More people started showing up with similar clarity and by that time it was pretty clear to me. If I could bring that clarity out from all the people I train and make them keep their eyes on it, it would greatly increase their chances of improving. And that's exactly what happened. Once they fully realised what was driving them they started caring more and more, which ultimately made them more focused and brought them the results they wanted. It was great.

MEANING BEHIND YOUR ACTION

Tom is a COO of an expanding company that sells water purifying machines. I've met about half a dozen people from their company and their mission and vibe are excellent. Even more than that, a lot of things are happening according to Tom. And man he's a dynamic person. He's 35, been busy with expanding the businesses globally and is now expecting a kid. He's never had a 6-

pack. His wife is due to go into labour in 3 months and from that point on he will be even busier taking care of his wife and baby so if he doesn't do it right now he's going to have to wait a few years or perhaps never get it at all. Given the circumstances, him not going for it right now means he might not get what he's always wanted in the back of his mind for a very long time. That is the meaning behind everything he does in the gym from now on. And he understands it perfectly, which gives him a lot of power day in day out and makes him excel. The next thing you know, he loses 3kg of bodyweight and 6% of his body fat, and gains a visible 6-pack in 2 months - a month earlier than planned. He is a great example of someone who's got a reason that he's connected with. Knowing this reason automatically puts a meaning behind his action.

HYPE NEVER LASTS

The meaning must be coming from your own reason though and not from anything else. The funny thing about fitness industry is the seasonal hype you get every January and February as a result of New Year's resolutions and in September when everyone realises they're a bit out of shape after summer holidays. Loads of people start talking about gym, about training, about food and everyone's mind is all of a sudden hyped on the idea of improving their bodies. Everyone goes for it for a few weeks and then the music stops. People change their focus back with nothing achieved at all. So that's not the kind of meaning and reason I'm talking about because hype never lasts. If you don't have a strong enough reason to do it any time of the year then don't expect to follow through because the crowd intensifies your focus for a while. It's unsustainable. If you want to make a change you need to be in touch with yourself and understand your game consistently. That's why you need to understand your genuine reasons for doing it. Hype is not enough. There have definitely been a few people who told me they were surprised by the value I assign to exploring and defining their reason but everyone found it absolutely revealing, empowering, and beneficial for their body transformation journeys. It's definitely worth your time and you definitely want it. If you're serious about training and pushing on all fronts you want a reality check every now and then to re-focus, re-calibrate and bring some clarity into your actions so you're confident you're not wasting your time.

CLIENT CONSULTATIONS

Consultations are how I normally explore people's reasons before I even start working with them. The first time I got consulted I was blown away. I thought I was on top of my game, sitting opposite my first gym manager, who was probably double my size, had a great charisma and looked like someone I could comfortably look up to. He'd been in the industry for a while and was definitely quality. We sat down so he could show me how to consult people his way and man he made me step my game up. It was so revealing. It not only made me re-focus on my training and diet but put me back on track the way I needed. No explanations needed, I learned it from him in few months after practising with numerous people who must have wondered what I was trying to get to on a few occasions. It was incredible. A well-led consultation can make a big difference in how you approach your training in terms of your motivation, attitude and connection you make on a deep level with your personality and your goals. It is the best way to get you in touch with yourself and help you define a reason that will make you move forward. It is a must and it's the most revealing experience you'll ever get within the gym environment.

THE HIDDEN VALUE

Sadly enough, consultations are probably the most under-utilised tool in the industry. It's an incredible tool for coaches to use and it's also absolutely critical for you to experience. A consultation will take you to a place of a different perspective, give you a snapshot of your fitness needs, establish your goals and lay out a systematic plan for you to improve and move on. It's an incredible opportunity for you to reflect on what you've done in the previous months, what's been working, what has not and to realistically evaluate your next move. It's incredibly powerful. You'll also reconnect from the perspective of your fitness to everything else you do and see if there are things that are more important to you or some things that are not important to you at all. Also remember that the most important thing for you is to establish your reasons for visiting the gym and working hard on yourself so you can push through and maxim your effort as much as possible. This is what the consultation is for. It's a time when you clearly state what you want from coming to the gym and how you're going to get it. It's not likely that you have time to think about things like this outside of these consultations anyway. You've got way too many things to think about in The City and if you think some occasional 2 minutes thinking about this before you go to sleep are the same then you've never been consulted properly.

EMOTIONS DRIVE BEHAVIOUR

So let's see what difference a consultation can make. Daniel is working out 3 times a week to get fitter but he hates running, cycling or doing any cardio based exercise so that makes it a bit of a challenge for him initially. He wants to get fitter for so many reasons and yet he would not work out that regularly for one reason that would stop him from making his move. He hates doing boring things in the gym. Unless that changes, his emotions about the gym will not put him into motion. Explained and understood he soon finds an engaging way that is incredibly hard as well and effective and gets fitter and happier while making his first breakthrough multimillion pound deal outside the gym at the age of 23. Think about the aftermath. Now all of this is possible because he's real about his reasons and is willing to share his expectations with me so I can personalise his experience as much as I possibly can so we're both controlling the session and working on it together rather than playing a master and a follower game.

Now that requires a certain level of trust but it is the best leverage we could ever use working together on his objectives. The point is that if you really want to change your body it's crucial that you find those reasons and leverage them as much as you can because it might be the difference between a deal maker and a deal breaker.

THE GOOD, THE BAD AND THE NASTY

So when you're exploring your reasons be honest about them. You're not in this to be a part of something or to fill your time with an activity. You're sorting something out. Whether it's your lack of self-esteem, your fear of a heart attack, your desire to be the best on the golf course or your desire to look attractive for a partner just be real about it. It is for you to understand and to exploit. Take that piece of motivation and make good use of it. Make it get you what you want. Pretending your pain doesn't exist is not going to sort you out. I've once consulted a lawyer who has only been to the gym twice in his life and he claimed he had no other reason for joining the gym than having it as a part of his routine for health. Now I know there's always something more than that but the story of his body transformation stays unwritten. So be real about your reasons and you'll fast track your way to your goals. Think about your motivations, know yourself and understand your desires.

JUDGING YOUR DRIVERS

The nature of what drives you doesn't matter as long as you understand it. I had someone telling me they wanted to look like Zac Efron about a year ago for whatever reason, but it was genuine and real. I saw them working really hard for a few months right after. Explore your drivers and be real about them. Your genuine understanding of yourself will help you get what it is that you want because it will give you power in the moments when you're tired and it's easy to slack off. Whether you're driven by the desire to always be complimented as the fittest person in the room or you're motivated by the desire to actual your performance potential I don't mind. As long as you're driven. You could be doing it for your health, for your therapy or simply out of vanity or a desire to be better than everyone else. It doesn't really matter that much as long as you're real about it. Don't disqualify your reasons. Nobody needs to know about them if you don't want to. If you want to have wide shoulders because you think it will make you look more masculine and you want that kind of look for whatever reason, then understand it and move on.

INSPIRATION OR DESPERATION

The last thing I want to touch on in this chapter is inspiration and desperation. I've once met a recruiter who told me: "Dreams don't sell anymore. Fear does mate." He had no problem understanding it because he was making money on it. Now my message to you is not to wait till you're desperate. It might be how you're wired initially but it's a self-destructive behaviour which makes no sense if you want to improve on something constructively. I've recently been watching a lot of people around me making changes in their lives. Not only working out in the gym but changing jobs, changing partners and even changing cities. Making a change is not easy. You need to have a reason. And the reason has to be fairly strong. But you don't need to wait to hit rock bottom to make your move. Don't wait for your doctor to tell you to lose weight because your thyroid is not functioning properly. Move on your own terms and move with your own initiative. Remember it's either inspiration or desperation and loads and loads of people are driven by desperation. Explore your reasons and make them empower you.

III. The perspective of fitness to your core values

MULTIDIMENSIONAL THINKING

This is where it gets interesting now because behind every reason there's another reason. And if you've been doing well without realising this then this will make you unstoppable. Chris was the first breakthrough client I had. He went from 70 kg to 76kg within his first 10 weeks while reducing his body fat by 2% and making new personal bests on many compound lifts which was definitely something to be proud of. Now not to forget, he did it because he wanted to get stronger and bigger at the time so it was a success. Instead of celebrating though I had a different challenge because I had two clients who were given the same tools but were showing very little to no progress. And so I came to Chris and asked him what made him follow through so I could help my non-performing clients make some progress. And not surprisingly it was his reason. But this time he told me about his deeper reason that was driving him on a more advanced level. He told me his cousin used to eat really badly and got diagnosed with cancer in his early 20s and then after being treated and told to improve on his nutrition he didn't change anything and got diagnosed again. At that point Chris decided to take great care of his body, train consistently and eat good and healthy foods so he would never be in his cousin's position himself. And that's what was going on in his mind on a deeper level. He made a connection with his reason and made it empower him. And with that power he could make a lasting change.

WHY DO I CARE ABOUT YOUR DEEPEST REASON?

Look, if your reason for working on your body is where the power is then I want you to be connected with it all the time the same way Chris was. It's difficult to make a connection with your goal of reducing your body fat by 5%. You need to connect with the deepest reason behind you wanting to lose those 5% of your body fat and even then you still need to maintain the connection. You might lose that connection every now and then as a busy City professional but it's my job not to let you. I want to figure out who you are as a person and coach you effectively. And I need to because I want to give you what you want – your results and everything that goes with it. Whether it's your improved lifestyle, confidence, self-esteem, job promotion, increase in sales, new contacts, wellbeing or happiness with your kids, I want you to have it all.

WHAT DOES LOOKING GOOD MEAN TO YOU?

So going into depth is imperative. Not only can you not make a connection with your reason but it's also that different people have different interpretations so the meaning of the words can be lost in communication. It's a very common thing for people to say they want to be fit. It seems to be a way of saying they want to look good. When I ask them what being fit means to them that's exactly what most of them tell me. "I want to look good." So what does looking good mean to you? It means to be able to wear all the clothes I want, having more definition and a little more size on my upper body. OK, why do you want more definition? Because I want this and this and this. Why do you want those? Because of this and this. I know I always sound tricky and difficult with these questions but I'm doing it to understand what people actually want. If we stopped at arriving to the conclusion that you want to be fit just for the sake of being fit, I would have had no idea that you actually wanted to get ready for your next beach holiday because you felt embarrassed on the last one. The point is this. I want to help you find your deepest reason so I understand where you're coming from and can get you in touch with it so you've got some power behind your action.

GETTING FIT OR BEING COMFORTABLE IN YOUR CLOTHES?

Understanding your deeper reason automatically raises your stakes and forces you to do something about your current state. Imagine going down from the office to a corner pub to have a pint with your colleagues and then imagine taking a cab and meeting someone to negotiate a multimillion pound contract. Now, the stakes are different so you'll make sure you're on that cab on time and ready to do what needs to be done whereas you might be more willing to compromise if it's just hanging out with your friends. You've got a stronger reason to follow through. That's what I'm trying to achieve with this reasoning. If we sit down and chat, I will always try to find your deepest reason for transforming your body because the deeper you get the stronger it is. And I guarantee you will not make any change if the stakes are small and your decisions don't carry any weight. And that's the key to achievement and a part of human behaviour that can be applied to your body transformation as well. It's always interesting to watch people train and see how much they care because the way they care is almost exclusively always directly related to the strength of their reason. Of course they've got different personalities but it's ultimately their focus on their reason that makes them move forward. Ability is never in question.

YOUR STAKES IN THIS

So once you real how your body influences your desires, experiences and outcomes on a deeper level your stakes will automatically increase. Not because the situation is different but because you understand the situation differently and more clearly. You'll see what things you're missing on when you're not treating your body the way you should. So if you're training because you're not comfortable with your body and want to increase your confidence or your self-esteem through training then a lack of training will not help your confidence and self-esteem too much and you'll miss certain opportunities when they arrive because you won't have the confidence to grab them and turn them into your wins. If you make solid progress though and your confidence and self-esteem go up you'll demand more things from life and when the same opportunities come you'll be ready to take control of them which can make a lot of difference. Now this is the tricky bit because most of the people who transformed their bodies under my coaching actually confessed that they couldn't see the impact on other things until those things actually started happening. So when I look back now I wish I could paint that picture to them back then. What you can't see in advance doesn't mean it's not there though and it's my duty and obligation to present it to you now. Do you believe your body transformation is only about your body or do you think it influences more things? If you stretch your imagination and believe in your ability to real your vision, you'll see the idea behind this paragraph.

WHAT ARE YOUR CORE VALUES?

At the end of 2014 I've started spending a lot of time with a high performance coach Tim Robinson. If you've never met Tim he is the type of person who is very enthusiastic about what he does and has no problem taking it to the extreme. When I first started in coaching he introduced me to the game and we became good friends. As our schedules matched a lot of the times it was easy for us to escape the rush of the day and talk about how to improve the experience for our clients, how to increase our ability to give them what they want and how to take our business to the next level. It has always been extremely important for us and it is one of the most important things we care about up to this day. We're always trying to provide the best service possible. Now in order to do that we need to understand our clients and in most cases we're successful because we manage to understand them down to their core values. Now, the point for you to take is that whether you believe you're motivated by money or you're driven by freedom or new experiences or anything else, you need to understand those core values too. Understanding those and then linking the progress you can make with your body to the progress it can potentially allow you to make with the subject of your core values is one of the major factors in your success.

WALKING WITH INTEGRITY

So what do I mean by your core values? There are 13 different core life values we mostly relate to on a personal level. Family, financial resources, friends, health & fitness, home, leadership, leisure pursuits, personal growth, public service, spirituality and work satisfaction. Now everyone might have a different hierarchy of those. The most important thing though is to know which ones are the most important to you and base your strategy around them. So if you're trying to work on your body and pretend it's the most important thing you need to do, while actually believing that it's the most pointless thing to do you won't feel fulfilled and you're likely to stop working on your body in the long run. However, if you work on your body with the understanding that your job is the most important thing for you and you train because you want to feel great to be able to persuade people on all levels, then that will empower you. You will follow through with your training because you're true to yourself and you're walking with integrity.

WHAT'S THE PERSPECTIVE OF FITNESS TO YOUR CORE VALUES?

Now this is extremely important. Your fitness doesn't need to be your number one priority for you to be able to make a change in your body as long as you understand it from the perspective of your core values. If your job requires you to perform on a high level for 50 hours a week, you travel at least twice a month and you're also planning on starting a family then you're not likely to worship the gym like you would in your early 20's. Let's be real. Your priorities are somewhere else. Your body is still incredibly important though. Position it from a different perspective. How can making progress with your body influence your ability to deliver to your clients or customers? Do you think your increased confidence, hormonal health and blood flow can influence it? Have you ever experienced the direct impact of your body performance on your mental performance? How can being in great shape help you with starting a family? Maybe you've got more energy to do everything? Maybe your partner is happier and more proud to be with you? There are loads of questions to be asked for you to see the correlation. The most important question though is this: Do you believe you can experience more quality with your priorities if you take care of your body? If you do, then keep on reading.

MAP OF DESIRES

You simply need to be in touch with yourself and your core values if you want to transform your body and step your game up. There have been numerous talks I've had with Tim and countless discussions on the topic of fitness and high performance and almost all of them basically lead to that same conclusion. You need to be connected to your core values. We've coached many people, tried lots of strategies, experienced lots of success as well as some failures but the ultimate knowledge we got out of it is incredible so we're able to get people into their zone. Now if you're a person of high ambition and high consciousness then you probably understand your incentives for doing things on many levels and it's incredibly important that you understand your incentives for getting into fitness as well so you can connect with them, get what you want and move on. Not everyone in the City is necessarily an expert on human biochemistry, nutrition and exercise but you can get people to coach you on those. The really important thing, if you're chasing a goal of body transformation in The City, is to actually follow through and do things the smart way so you see your results. The reward is attractive and the price is worth your hustle more than anything else.

WHY YOU MUST SEE THE BIG PICTURE

Once you understand how your progress influences what matters the most to you you can nicely position it in your big picture and put it onto your roadmap. It's time to stop looking at the gym as a separate thing you do for your health. Look at it from the perspective of what's important to you. If you want to be a leader in your community, then you definitely want to be in the zone so your community sees you're on top of your game as a person of vision, making things happen all the time. If you want to make an impression on people because of your job or your social life, then it's easier to present yourself as a person who takes care of themselves rather than a person of poor health. If you're trying to raise your confidence because you're constantly pitching someone on a daily basis, then it's incredibly important to have an optimal hormonal balance. Your body simply belongs to that picture. You know what you want and you know what your big picture looks like so make sure your body has its place in there.

PATRICK

The perfect person to demonstrate this is Patrick. I could call him an ambassador for Sets In The City. He makes massive progress in his first few months, gets promoted with his company, enjoys massive dating success and makes every group of people he gets in contact with feel great because of his energy. Things are great and it's time to celebrate. But then he changes his focus, his progress slows down and he slowly plateaus over the next few weeks. It's just what naturally happens. So one day he comes to the gym and we're looking together for some new answers to find out why he's plateauing. "I guess I'm not pushing hard anymore and consider things to only be a part of my routine now." I make him remember the greatest moments of all the events that happened while he was seeing progress, he reconnects with his reasons for training and he rips the gym apart in the following 60 minutes and gets back to top of his game soon after. He's the greatest example of everything this chapter is about. The degree to which he can connect to his drivers and his core values now makes a dramatic difference to what he's doing with his body and to all the things that are influenced by its impact.

TOP GAME MOTIVATION

So the question is how do you keep your motivation on the highest level all the time? So many people I train with have been constantly getting into the zone and pushing to the limit when they need to. I call it the top game motivation and it is the same zone you get into when you're facing a tough deadline or a fine or you're about to close an important deal. You know exactly what the stakes are and what the rules are and you give it your best to come victorious at the moment that counts. You understand every single reason and you've got to make it happen. There's no other option. Top game motivation. What I want to accomplish in this book is to take that moment, take your mindset and apply it to your body. I've already described my reasons for doing it and I've also already described the reasons for you doing it so now it's only up to you to decide what you're going to take out of it. Remember there's a reason why you're paying for your gym membership and there's also a reason why you're reading this book. And behind those reasons are deeper reasons that lead to your core values which you can't trick.

YOUR VISION

This had all been around for a while and most people already understand it these days. Although it's all been very blurred. I'm now sitting opposite to an old friend of mine. The last time we saw each other was almost 2 years ago and so we're catching up in a pub. He just got back from Australia after 9 months and has a plan to roll out back here in London. The product needs to be created, the website done and some good contacts gained. All in 10 weeks which is a tough job indeed. The first thing to be done though is joining the gym. Primarily to strengthen his game. And that's what he plans to starts with. Now this is an interesting thing because the connection between working on your body and strengthening your inner game is not a new concept anymore. Everyone who's ever worked on their body and gained momentum discovered the impact on their mental health and performance as well. Now the question is whether or not you're forgetting about it because if you're constantly stretching yourself to get to the new level you can always give yourself an edge by starting with your body.

CAN YOU FACE YOUR CONSCIOUSNESS?

All of this is basically about making the connection with your deep reasons for your fitness goals so you take action. I've seen people changing their bodies and I've seen people who wanted to change but never did and the difference was that people who changed their body got so many extra bonuses and rewards from life compared to people that didn't and stayed in their comfort zone questioning their ability or timing or whatever was holding them back. Again, we're in the City so I don't expect you to devote half a day each day to working out and dieting. But you can definitely transform your body with the busy schedule you've got if you're a bit smart about it. Every day you make a choice to either treat or not treat your body the way you should and if you don't then you have to be ready to pay the price. And the price in this case is accepting that you'll never be able to overcome those reasons you defined as the driving force behind the thoughts you've got for your body in the first place. So if you want to be fit to support your self-esteem or you want to look good for dating or you want to be able to keep up with your kids as they grow up then the time to do something about it is now. Next chapter will tell you how to go around it in The City where you're busy 24/7.

IV. Doing things The City way

THE HUSTLE GROUND

You're called into a meeting where you learn you need to create a presentation and fly out to pitch a new prospect on a tight deadline. Then you receive a text from someone inviting you to an event you definitely need to go to and then you come home and your fridge is empty because you've been busy doing all kinds of things unrelated to taking care of your body. The last two chapters were about how to gain some power behind what you do with your body so you've got a body your partner likes, you can join your colleagues on a cycle to Paris or you can increase your confidence to successfully manage your pipeline. Now the question of this chapter is about the long-term high performance sustainability in the environment that we all share here in The City. The hustle environment. How do you stay on top of your game? That's the focus of this chapter. I've tried to stay pretty consistent with The City all throughout the book so now let's take a look at why.

A TYPICAL CITY AGENDA

Your schedule is always fully loaded, your business requires networking and drinking, you're commuting to your office and travelling to other countries for business, the food around is not ideal, beer is everywhere around and your social life is pretty extensive. There are times when you can't go down to the gym or eat what you ideally need to eat. There are also times when you have a pint and it's not just one and there are times when you're under stress that takes up a lot of your focus. That's what happens in The City and that's what's normal which is why you need to work on your body The City way. Your objective is to make a choice about your breakfast, a choice about your drinks when the situation allows you not to touch them, a choice about your training and your visits to the gym and your choice about your commitment to the vision you've established with your body. You have to play along with The City and still stay on top of your game.

WHY IS IT HARD TO STAY ON TOP OF YOUR GAME?

A brilliant question to ask someone in M&A. I've had the chance to train with a few of them and their workload is a bit crazy. Same as some other people. If you work 300 to 350 hours a month, it's easy to lose it. Let's keep it real. The first thing on your mind might be some rest and the second some fun or social activity. So unless you keep selling yourself on your need to take care of your body you're very likely to be losing your focus. Now we've already been through fitness economics so you should understand the value of taking care of your body. Clearly dropping your gym activity is not an option, which means you need to be on top of your game whenever you have the chance to pay attention. Otherwise you come to the gym, have no steam, no drive, no system and therefore no results which then becomes pointless. You stop seeing the value and you're out. Losing your time and wasting your potential to sort out whatever got you there in the first place. Back to square one. Remember you want something out of it. Your high ambitions in life mean you need to be smarter about it which is what this book is about.

DO YOU HAVE HIGH EXPECTATIONS ABOUT EVERYTHING?

High expectations about your career, about your social circle, about your family, about your romance, about your holidays, nights out, experiences, education, finance, hobbies and so many other things. Now the point is that they're not in a conflict of interest with your body objectives. Think about each and every one of them as a support for each other. "I know I would lose weight if I stopped boozing." The most common fitness sentence in The City. You can lose weight while boozing. I've seen it happening many times. Positioning these two as something that can't happen at the same time is a rookie mistake. You might need to reduce and plan your boozing but in reality it's possible. "I can't make any progress with my body because I travel for work too much." There must be a gym in a hotel where you stay. All my clients have always managed to find the time to find a gym and have a workout when they're traveling so I know it's possible. Think about your expectations of multiple areas of your life as each supporting the other ones and positioning them in a place of conflict will not appear attractive and constructive to you anymore.

HADRIEN'S VIEW

Hadrien's had great progress in the last 3 months so we're reflecting on what we've done and chatting a bit when he's got a remarkable statement. For someone who's never seriously committed to their body, it might seem a bit impossible to do that in the rush of The City with the idea that they would need to stop their social lives, live in the gym instead and completely change their lifestyle to serve their gymming needs. The reality is different though, which actually surprises him. Still hanging out with his friends, partying almost every weekend, focusing properly on his job and making investment decisions, he's able to shed 6kg of bodyweight in 3 months by being smart about it. Now that still takes some sacrifice but his case, as loads of other people's cases, only prove that getting results is completely achievable within your possibilities and your commitments in The City if you do things the smart way. And that's what the most impressive thing is. You can transform your body while keeping your busy City life without sacrificing everything else.

DON'T LIVE IN THE GYM, MAXIMISE YOUR EFFORTS

So if you're hustling all the time you need to be very smart about your body and the way you're taking care of it. Your workouts need to be tailored to your needs, your food plan needs to cater for your busy schedule and your focus needs to be good enough for you to follow through. A programme suitable for an average person is not going to work for you as a busy City professional. You won't find steamed cod with sweet potatoes and greens at every corner. Your client lunches and dinners are going to happen as business is about people so you need to cater for that as well. You'll find yourself in a hotel where all they've got are 3 treadmills and a weights room smaller than your living room. Your circumstances are extraordinary so your approach to your body needs to respond to that. Learn to maxim with your body. The same way you maxim your trading decisions by heavily leveraging on them, maxim your body by leveraging on the smart things you can do within your busy daily agenda. You need to take care of your body if you want to perform on a top level and with the time and focus you can afford to give it you want to make sure you're doing it right.

ONLY CARING ABOUT COACHING

The first time I found out what power The City really had was when I started training an Australian investment banker. He's working insane hours, doing business globally and travelling around Europe whenever he can. He loves working out hard and it's easy training with him but his eating habits are completely upside down. He's eating only one massive meal a day, snacking around it and drinking beer 2-3 days a week. Now of course he doesn't feel great about it and has the intention of improving it but the reality is different. He starts by having 2 meals a day and having breakfast. It's a bit of a struggle initially but then he gets into it so after 4 weeks we make another step and that's to have 3 meals a day – breakfast, lunch and dinner. After 2 weeks I ask him if he's doing dinners and he tells me he is now 4 times a week which is great. But then I ask him if he's still doing breakfast and he's not anymore. He says he hasn't got any time for it. Now I've seen him coming back from some holidays and I know he can do it if he's not pressured with work but having to work is somewhat of a block for him. This is the influence of The City.

THE CITY DIET

Everyone knows what it looks like. 3 meals a day, a packet of crisps and a few pints on some days when you're out with your friends, colleagues or your clients. Now out of those 3 meals a day one is a sandwich with some sugary drink and perhaps some chocolate or something sweet instead of crisps. A coffee a day is not working for most of the people anymore and so working without any caffeine is something never heard of. Now it might be a lot better or a lot worse but imagine how your body feels about it. All this food has a massive influence on your looks, on your fitness, on the way you feel about your body, on your performance and on the outcome of your micro-situations. I know that the food around is not ideal but unfortunately that's what eating in the City is like so when we go back to your objectives we need to remember this. Now the point of this is to remind you of your eating as it's nothing new but again it's something that you might fall for because it's convenient. There are options for you in the City and you don't need to eat salads all day long to get what you want. I've had clients who I know have not dropped drinking all throughout their transformation but because the combination of their food, drinking and training was well-timed they managed to change their bodies, get awesome results and enjoy themselves all along as well. It's just being real about it within the options and desires you naturally have.

SOCIAL LIFE IN THE CITY

So after the diet there is also the social life issue that might seemingly clash with your body transformation plans. You could easily spend all day every day just networking. Making plans, shaking hands and following up on the promises to people around you and to yourself. You might have a partner, mastermind group or a close inner circle you see on a regular basis and all of this is necessary but takes up your time. You might expect to drink with loads of people, follow them to certain places and events and have a normal City social life. Now the idea is not to take this away from you because it would make absolutely no sense. Your social life is a part of what you do. Nothing happens without people and you need to take a good care of them. The idea is to allow you to keep your busy social life and still manage to take care of your body in a way that makes you feel great because you're making some real progress. With that progress you feel better and you project it in all your social interactions as well, which makes people feel safe about you which is a big win for you again. Don't perceive fitness as an obstacle for your social life, see it as a booster.

WHAT'S STU DOING?

13 stag dos and weddings with most of them out of country and all within 4 months. Now if you think about Stu's already busy work and social life it is incredible how he commits to his improved health and lifestyle despite his crazy schedule. So what's happening? I'm meeting Stu about a month before it all starts. We're fully set for his fat loss and definition programme and we're getting a bit of momentum when the first event comes. Miami. Expect the damage. So he comes back, gets into a rhythm, things are going well and then another event arrives. Great fun, loads of good memories but zero progress. Now at this stage it's pretty clear to both of us – we 're not going to reach his original goals. His weekends are pretty much all spent abroad and he's packing the things he would normally do over the weekend into his already busy working days which all means he can commit to 2 workouts a week maximum and is not going to get what he wants. Now this is a very important moment because he's making a decision. He could easily say you know what, I'm extremely busy so let's forget about it and I'll only come back to the gym when it's all finished. Instead he commits to coming twice a week and gives it everything he's got so when this all ends he's ready to go all in and get what he wants. He's weathering the storm. And

that's exactly what happens. His global stag do and wedding tour ends and he's on top of his game. Sometimes it's extremely challenging to follow what you want but it definitely can be done.

MEETING GLYN IN A PUB

Now I already mentioned beer is the drink of choice in The City and I've got an interesting story to tell. So I happen to be in a pub in the area around New Year's and my client Glyn walks in with his colleagues for a pint after a successful day in business. They're in the busiest phase of the year as most of their clients renew their contracts right around January and so it's time to for them to hang out a bit after work. Now we're both in a pub with a few people and so we merge groups for a moment and have a pint together. And while I encourage people to cut down on booze I also understand that beer is the drink in the City and everyone working here will have a pint every now and then. So we have one together. But let me tell you about Glyn now. He's got 2 children, had a hip replacement surgery a few years ago, and from not being able to do any sports or activity before or after his surgery, he's now able to do a 3-minute plank, 5 pull-ups, cycle to Brighton, train 4-5 times a week and get to his best bodyweight in the last 11-12 years. So although beer might not be a part of fitness lifestyle it is a part of The City fitness lifestyle and what really matters, is that although everyone might have a pint in The City every now and then, working on your body and getting your results is possible if you're on top of your game and pay attention to what's important.

FITNESS AS A PART OF LIFESTYLE

All of these things are a part of what makes living in The City of London special. They affect every ambitious person and so we need to learn how to do more while living here. And I know it is possible. During the time I'm writing this book I've had the best progress with my body in the last 2 years. I'm busy too. 24/7. But I know that a connection of multiple little streams creates a powerful river. So fitness must become a part of your lifestyle if you want to move forward as powerful as possible for all the reasons you've identified and understand as they're your own. Even with the constraints of The City. This book is about making that progress with your body towards the goals you set up for yourself so you can excel in everything else as well. If you're not working on your body at the moment or you haven't had any progress last 6 months, it's like missing one of those streams, which leads to a loss of your personal power. Not too great for any power player.

WHAT DOES TRAINING MEAN TO YOU NOW?

I hope you can see your body and fitness from a different perspective. It's your journey towards your confidence on the beach, towards your confidence in front of your partner, it's your way of keeping up with your kids, it's your ritual for projecting safety and trust in your body language, it's your way of not collapsing every time you climb a few stairs, it's something more than just training and it's all super tailored from the position of a busy City hustler. The meaning it holds for you is hidden behind many why's you need to ask yourself. Understand those why's and make them empower you. The City life is very special and has its own way of almost dictating your lifestyle but link the meaning of training to everything that makes your City life happy and you'll find the drive to go through your body transformation and take your life to the next level. All of what this really is about is to how to maximise your motivation 24/7/365. How do you make yourself follow up on your decision to lose 5kg when The City steals your focus unless you double protect it? Combining your goals and reasons with The City life and making it work in whatever circumstances you're in is something we can all do. Meetings, travels, events, friends, family, personal goals or whatever your ambitions and core values are all worth the benefits you get from leveraging on your City life and making some solid progress with your body.

V. Winners' hall

WHY CITY PEOPLE GO TO GYM AND TRAIN

Answering this question has been one of the main goals for this book and I hope my message is clear. There's so much more to it than just coming in and training and that's why it's important that you take the message from this book and think about what's really driving you, what your reasons for taking care of your body are and how it affects your core values and the things that are most important to you. Look, whether it's your career, your relationship, romance, the way you come across with people, your ability to enjoy your holidays or anything else important to you, having your optimal body can help you reach it in a way your current body can't at the moment. There are doors opening for the people that push through and make progress with their body as a ripple effect because they get into a completely different mindset that helps them get what they want. Their hormonal balance changes, their ability to focus and be present in the moment improves and their inner game tightens up. These people live and work in the City just like you and they're living the message of this book right as you read it. You've already seen some of their stories and I'm going to show you more because stories are how we ultimately remember important information and the stories you're about to read reveal important messages.

PATRICK'S SUCCESS

So I've already described a part of Patrick's story. He wants to put some muscle on as he's quite tall and 78kg looks rather skinny on him. As soon as he starts seeing some results he pushes even more as it's a kind of a self-motivating thing for him. He makes massive progress in his first few months, gets promoted with his company, enjoys dating success and makes every group of people he gets in contact with feel great. People are seeing his results and compliment him all the time. Now the thing that's interesting about his story is that he's in this for the long term but he's got phases where he's inconsistent. It might be because he's a salesman or because he's got a large group of people to hang out with or because his agenda is always packed. But for whatever reason there's always a time when he goes 5 days without a workout at least once every 3 months. But when he's consistent he works out hard, cooks his food and takes good care of his body. Which proves one simple concept. Your agenda might sometimes not let you maintain laser focus on everything at the same time but you can at least achieve laser focus on whatever your agenda has for you at the time.

JAMES' SUCCESS

James has a great story too. He wants to lose some weight and run faster because he wants to upgrade his appearance and having young kids means he wants to be fit enough to keep up with them as well. Although he's been doing distance running for a few years his bodyweight has never really changed. But then he notices one of his friends getting great results with a trainer and decides to give it a try. Now 12 weeks go by and he's gone from 86kg to 79kg, which is his 10-year best. He's already achieved his best time ever on a 10K run as well, got promoted and is now expecting a baby with his wife. Things are great. Now having already achieved all of that, he's not finished yet and is hungry for more instead of becoming complacent, and so we set up a new challenge and go for his 20-year best which is 76kg, while he also sets up a new measurement for fitness which is to hold a plank for longer than it takes to finish a 1k row on a rowing machine. The first time he tries doing both he gets 3:47 on rowing and 3:24 on a plank and he ultimately beats it 2 weeks after when he holds his plank for 5 minutes straight. The ultimate transformation story.

CHRIS' SUCCESS

I've already touched on Chris' story as well when I described his deeper reason for working on his body in one of the previous chapters but there's still more to learn. The training with him is about being strong and being fit as he's constantly sitting in his office as a lawyer and wants to stay fully functional and good-looking. However, his circumstances only allow him to commit to 3 days of training a week. His goal is clear. He wants to put some lean size on with those 3 days a week available. And he's aiming for about 5kg of size within 3 months. Now 10 weeks go by, he's put on 6kg already, had to buy new clothes as his old shirts are tight, has beaten all of his old personal bests on deadlifts, squats, bench press, lat pulldowns and military press and has been so impressed by his own progress that he's referred his girlfriend to me as well. He's packed on 6kg of size while his body fat percentage stayed the same and he did it with 3 workouts a week. Two workouts on Tuesdays and Thursdays at 7am and one workout on Saturdays with me. Now the point of his story is to tell anyone who thinks they've got no time to do it that it can be done and this proves it completely.

GARETH'S SUCCESS

Strength, fitness, muscle mass and definition. We've been through a lot in the time we've trained together. Gareth comes from a rugby background and hasn't trained properly in ages due to a shoulder problem, knee surgery and a hernia, and is now trying to get back into training, lose a bit of weight, keep his workouts fresh and ultimately play one more game of rugby when his time comes. He's working around the corner, is a decision-maker and lives a busy City life. He's committed to working out and has always enjoyed it so it's something to really look forward to. We set up goals and start working on them and he goes from 60kg deadlifts with poor form to 160kg deadlifts with perfect form in a little less than 10 months, manipulating his bodyweight in both ways during the same time and increasing his fitness from

10 minutes of tough high intensity training to 40 minutes on extremely difficult intervals. Now although it's most likely some muscle memory contributing to Gareth's jump you don't see results like his happening every day which makes it worth sharing.

ROB'S SUCCESS

Rob's been the most determined and enthusiastic person I've ever had the pleasure to train with. His transformation story starts when he moves to London to do some asset management for one of the biggest organizations in the UK. He's exchanged a few years of his life for money in the mining industry and is now ready to clean up all the impact it has had on his body. He starts at 126kg, and is initially aiming for double-digits while his brother and one his friends have already lost an incredible amount of weight. Along with some other reasons he's got for his transformation he wants to join their success. Now it takes him 1 month to shed his first 10kg and another few months to get to 108kg which is almost 20kg of weight loss. The interesting thing is what happens next. He plateaus and he plateaus big time and stays at the same number for a bit over 2 months. It's not easy for him to break through as he's eating a lot of protein in the first place to protect as much muscle as possible during his transformation but now with some beers on top it's incredibly hard for him unless he goes to back to his original eating habit. He flies back home to Australia for holidays, puts on a little more weight, bounces back to 113kg, flies back, takes a deep breath and is now on his way to two digits, within the next few weeks. It takes him another 2 months but he hits his double-digit goal and celebrates big time.

A SUCCESS WRAP UP

So it is important to note here, that while all these stories are a bit different with different lessons to learn, all success has something in common. With all the top achievers mentioned in this book it is their ability to define their reasons for transforming their body that ultimately allows them to make the impressive and lasting change they are looking for. They've got the same tools as a lot of people but get results other people can only dream of. Jason's ultimately loses 22kg in 5 months and is now enjoying a fitter and healthier life, Priya goes from 59kg to 54kg in the preparations for her wedding and will forever be happy when she looks at her wedding photos, Gareth's become one of the strongest and fittest people in the gym and is now considering playing rugby again after many injuries from the previous years, and there are so many more I could mention and probably fill this page with. The most important thing though is that they clearly defined their reasons that ultimately allowed them to follow through and get what they wanted. Their success was not an accident and whatever else they got from life during those days was not an accident either.

IT'S NOT A CHOICE IT'S A NECESSITY

It all starts with defining what you want and more importantly why you want it. It is the only way you can have a connection with your goal and keep your eyes on it so you succeed in reaching your targets and improving the quality of your life. The connection is important because it's really easy to lose your mindset and start floating in the space if you don't know why you're hustling all day long trying to get things you're not connected to. If you want to change your body, this connection is a must. If you don't know why you're trying to get it then you don't know the consequences of not getting it, and you won't really understand the importance of you getting it. And that means your chances of getting it are automatically halved. It's so important to establish your reason. It gives you power. It gets you in the zone and gives you the drive. The essential drive that makes people work in the City, live in the City and spend their most important commodity, time, on something that is bigger than them – their vision.

THE OPPORTUNITY COST

And what happens if you don't build the connection and don't manage to step up? There's a price to pay. So what's the price for you? Seemingly you could say nothing really happens if you don't take care of your body on a top level because your body might stay the same or get a bit worse but you'll be fine. But is it so? Is it not true that by not changing the thing you want to change on your body, the original reason will stay with you as your roadblock to certain other things you want to do? Would it not be great for you to free yourself from it so you can expand into new activities or experiences you've never had? If you want to lose weight because you want to be a great parent and keep up with your kids, then not doing it bears the price of you sitting in a chair or standing on the spot while your kids want to play some sports with you or just joke around and you can't because you're out of breath really quickly. There's always price to pay. Things never stay the same. They get worse because you're cutting yourself off from what you really want. That's the price you pay and that's the opportunity cost.

THIS IS WHAT I PROMOTE

So as you're at the end of the book remember that all these insights come from my daily experience and observations. It took me a while to figure out how to get people to follow through but in the process I managed to clearly define what works and what I stand for. Do as much business as you can, hustle hard and make some serious money because all the desires you've got in your life and all the things you want to do and experience are going to cost you something. Whether you want to party in Ibiza or you want to sponsor education in a 3rd world country you will need money. Have an extensive social circle as people are what makes your life worthwhile. If it means going out and spending loads of time with them, it will not be a roadblock to what you want. Play hard, have fun, have the experiences, travel the world and go crazy because life is short and you only ever regret things you've never done.

But hey, doing all of this, make sure you're taking great care of your body. Your body is one of the most important things you've got and it can either make or break you. There's more to working on your body than just its appearance, fitness and functionality. It influences everything you do and it influences your core values and your personality so taking great care of it is not a choice. It's a necessity. And that's what I stand for.

HALO EFFECT

Patrick once told me about the concept of the halo effect, which is a cognitive bias in which an observer's overall impression of a person, company, brand, or product influences the observer's feelings and thoughts about that entity's character or properties, where positive feelings in one area cause ambiguous or neutral traits to be viewed positively as well. Now in normal words, if you're on a roll and other people see it they will without realising open new doors for you because everything they see about you is a little enhanced. Now your body is the first step to this halo effect. Imagine you're making great progress. Your mood goes up, your posture changes, your energy levels change and the perception of you as a person changes. That all sends a certain message to people through the way you conduct yourself. They see it, know you're on a roll and so they open up to an interaction with you. Next thing you know they introduce you into a new project where you meet new players and money comes along. Or they introduce you to new friends and you find a new partner. Or you get some discounts for merchandise or you get an invitation into an exclusive event or whatever.

WHAT ARE YOU WAITING FOR?

I'm calling for you to put the halo effect at work for you. This book is the legacy of my last 18 months. I wrote it not only to show you what everyone else in the industry is missing but to set it as a philosophy and a brand that you can relate to as a professional hustling in one of the greatest places on this planet offering opportunities to fuel your ambition. A brand that can represent people pushing through in their professional lives and working on their body at the same time. Something that connects the ambition with the uniqueness of the life in The City and allows you think about your body from a different perspective so you can enjoy the great benefits of your body together with all the bonuses progressing with your body naturally brings. There's a reason why people train and there's also a reason behind that reason that is very deep. Your body transformation lies within your core values.

CALL ME MAYBE?

Sets In The City is the brand I personally stand behind. I take interest in people and service them according to who they are in their core so I give them the results they want with their body. I train with high performance, high power City professionals who have ambition, drive, self-motivation and like to work hard and play hard. More importantly I help create stories. Stories about people who I've had the opportunity to work with and make their body transformations a reality. You can be my next story. I want to thank you for taking the time for reading my book and extend you an invitation to a consultation, to help you find out what training can mean for you and how this philosophy can become a part of your lifestyle. Call me or email me now and I will personally make sure you get the most from your fitness efforts you possibly can. See you soon.

Cheers

Vlad Galbavy
setsinthecity.co.uk
vlad@setsinthecity.com
0756 516 8324
linkedin: /Vlad Galbavy

"I have been training with Vlad for the last 6 months and through his guidance I have been able to achieve the lowest weight of the last 3-4 years. This book shows you exactly why."

Diego M.

"Vlad enables you to be better. As soon as I let go of my old presumptions and committed to doing things Vlad's way, the results started coming in."

Robert S.,
Asset Management Specialist

"I have been working with Vlad for over 18 months now, having started with him at a point where my fitness level had deteriorated and weight increased after many years of little dedicated exercise partly due to requiring a hip replacement some years ago. We set goals and have undertaken a varied and challenging programme combining weight orientated training with high intensity sessions. Despite my City lifestyle and diet not being entirely helpful, not only has my weight improved to a reasonable degree, but my general level of fitness and feeling of wellbeing have increased immeasurably. I now am much more active away from the gym, and taking on cycling challenges that I would not even have considered a few years ago. With Vlad my training is not a chore, and sometimes almost enjoyable, and when I am flagging he boosts my spirits with the odd bottle of slivovitz!"

Glyn Hall,
Divisional Director at BMS Re at BMS Group

For more success stories and video testimonials please visit
setsinthecity.co.uk